Anti-Inflammatory Diet for Beginners

Lose Weight Fast, Optimize Health, Slow Aging, Fight Inflammation, Conquer Pain & Increase Energy with the Anti-Inflammation Diet Recipes

Emma Rose

Table of Contents

Introduction

I want to thank you and congratulate you for purchasing the book, "Anti-Inflammatory Diet for Beginners: Lose Weight Fast, Optimize Health, Slow Aging, Fight Inflammation, Conquer Pain & Increase Energy with the Anti-Inflammation Diet Recipes."

This book is a compilation of anti-inflammation recipes that will help you lose excess weight fast and slow the body's aging process so you will always feel at your best the whole day. These recipes are also recommended by professionals to fight inflammation to prevent any complications associated with this condition. Also, you can use these recipes to help boost your energy for optimal health.

In this book, you will find recipes for breakfast, lunch, dinner, and dessert that you can mix and match to design your own meal plan. Aside from being anti-inflammatory, these recipes can also be used for other special diets like paleo and gluten-free diet.

Thanks again for purchasing this book, I hope you enjoy it! Please take some time to stop by and LIKE our Facebook page:

https://www.facebook.com/joypublishing

With gratitude,

Emma Rose

Chapter 1: The Basics of The Anti-Inflammatory Diet

Chronic inflammation has been tagged as one of the root causes of severe illnesses including most cancers and heart attack. Inflammation is a natural reaction of the body when it needs to heal an infection or injury. However, when inflammation occurs for no particular reason, it destroys the body and eventually causes illness.

Chronic inflammation is caused by excessive exposure to toxins, stress, genetic predisposition, lack of exercise, and unhealthy diet. Since diet plays a big role in containing this condition, it is important to learn how to choose the right food to reduce the risk of diseases especially in the long-term.

The Anti-Inflammatory diet is not intended to help the person lose weight or to follow a strict diet plan. It is more of a guide to choose the right foods so the body stays in its optimal state. Aside from preventing inflammation, this diet also provides vitamins, dietary fiber, minerals, and other nutrients for steady energy.

General Tips for Anti-Inflammatory Diet

1. Try different varieties of food each meal.

2. Incorporate as much fresh foods into each meal.

3. Minimize consumption of fast food and processed food.

4. Eat vegetables and fruits every day.

5. Consume between 2,000 to 3,000 calories each day. If you are less active, you will need lesser calories.

6. 50% of your calorie intake should come from carbohydrates, 30% should come from fat and 20% should come from protein.

7. Drink more water or, if not, choose beverages that contain mostly water like fruit juices and tea.

8. Purify your drinking water.

Chapter 2: Breakfast Recipes

Cherry Quinoa Porridge

Ingredients:

- ✓ 1 cup of water
- ✓ ½ cup of dried unsweetened cherries
- ✓ ½ cup of dry quinoa
- ✓ ½ tsp of vanilla extract
- ✓ 1 tbsp of honey
- ✓ ¼ tsp of ground cinnamon

Procedure:

1. Prepare a medium-sized saucepan and set it over medium-high heat. Then, add in the water, dry quinoa, unsweetened cherries, vanilla extract, and ground cinnamon. Stir the ingredients together then bring the mixture to a boil.

2. Reduce the heat then place the lid on the saucepan. Let it simmer for 15 minutes or until the quinoa is tender and all the liquid has been absorbed.

3. Drizzle with honey then serve.

Raspberry Green Tea Smoothie

Ingredients:

- ✓ 1 ½ cups of chilled green tea

- ✓ 1 banana

- ✓ 2 cups of frozen raspberries (unsweetened)

- ✓ 1 tbsp of honey

- ✓ ¼ cup of protein powder

Procedure:

1. In a blender, add in the chilled green tea and honey. Combine the liquids together. Then, add in the banana, unsweetened raspberries, and protein powder. Blend until the mixture becomes smooth.

Gingerbread Oatmeal

Ingredients:

- ✓ 1 cup of water
- ✓ ¼ cup of dried and unsweetened cherries OR cranberries
- ✓ ½ cup of old-fashioned oats
- ✓ 1 tsp of ground ginger
- ✓ ¼ tsp of ground nutmeg
- ✓ ½ tsp of ground cinnamon
- ✓ 1 tbsp of flaxseeds
- ✓ 1 tbsp of molasses

Procedure:

1. Prepare a small saucepan and set it over medium-high heat. Add in the water, old-fashioned oats, unsweetened cherries or cranberries, ground ginger, ground cinnamon, and ground nutmeg. Stir the ingredients together. Bring the mixture to a boil then reduce the heat and simmer for 5 more minutes or until almost all of the liquid has been absorbed.

2. Add in the flaxseeds then cover the pan. Set it aside for 5 minutes.

3. Drizzle with molasses then serve.

Ginger Apple Muffins

Ingredients:

- ✓ 2 cups of all-purpose flour
- ✓ 1 tbsp of baking powder
- ✓ 2/3 cup of sugar
- ✓ ½ tsp of salt
- ✓ 1 tsp of ground ginger
- ✓ 1 tsp of ground cinnamon
- ✓ ¾ cup of unsweetened almond milk
- ✓ ½ cup of mashed ripe banana
- ✓ 1 cup of shredded apple
- ✓ 1 tbsp of apple cider vinegar
- ✓ ½ cup of finely chopped crystallized ginger

Procedure:

1. Turn on the oven and set it to 400F. Prepare a muffin pan with 12 cups and spray it with cooking spray or line it with paper liners.

2. In a large mixing bowl, add in the all-purpose flour, baking powder, sugar, ground cinnamon, salt, and ground ginger. Whisk the ingredients together until properly combined.

3. In a separate bowl, add in the unsweetened almond milk, apple, banana, apple cider vinegar, and crystallized ginger. Stir the ingredients together then gradually add in the flour mixture while stirring. Mix until the ingredients are well-incorporated. Fill the muffin cups with the batter about 2/3 of the way.

4. Place the muffin pan in the oven and bake for 15 minutes or until the muffins are done. To check, just insert a toothpick into the center of the muffin and, if it comes out clean, you'll know it's done.

Buckwheat and Quinoa Granola

Ingredients:

- ✓ 3 tbsp of honey

- ✓ 1 tsp of vanilla extract

- ✓ 3 tbsp of liquid coconut oil

- ✓ ¼ tsp of ground cinnamon

- ✓ 1 cup of buckwheat groats

- ✓ ¼ tsp of ground ginger

- ✓ 1 cup of cooked quinoa

- ✓ ½ cup of dried cranberries (unsweetened)

- ✓ ½ cup of old-fashioned oats

Procedure:

1. Turn on the oven and set it to 325F. Prepare a baking sheet and spray it with cooking spray or line it with parchment paper. You can also use a silicon baking mat if you have one.

2. In a bowl, add in the honey, liquid coconut oil, vanilla extract, ground cinnamon, and ground ginger. Stir the ingredients together until properly combined. In a larger bowl, add in the buckwheat groats, cooked quinoa, and old-fashioned oats. Stir then add in the honey mixture. Mix

until the ingredients are thoroughly combined. Spread the mixture onto the baking sheet and spread it evenly.

3. Place the baking sheet into the oven and bake for 40 minutes or until the grains are beginning to brown. Remove the pan from the oven then stir in the dried unsweetened cranberries. Place the baking sheet on a cooling rack and let it cool down completely before you store it in a tightly sealed container.

Spinach and Mushroom Frittata

Ingredients:

- ✓ 1 lb of button mushrooms, sliced
- ✓ 1 tbsp of freshly chopped garlic
- ✓ 1 large onion, chopped
- ✓ 1 lb of fresh spinach
- ✓ 6 large egg whites
- ✓ ¼ cup of water
- ✓ 4 large eggs
- ✓ ½ tsp of ground turmeric
- ✓ 5 oz of firm tofu
- ✓ ½ tsp of kosher salt
- ✓ ½ tsp of freshly cracked black pepper

Procedure:

1. Turn on the oven and set it to 350F.

2. Prepare a 10" ovenproof nonstick skillet or sauté pan and spray it with cooking oil. Set the pan over medium-high heat then sauté the mushrooms until they are golden brown. Add in the onion and cook for 3 minutes or until the onion is tender. Add in the garlic and cook for 30

seconds. Add in the water and spinach then place a lid on the pan. Cook for 2 minutes or until the spinach is wilted. Then, remove the lid and continue cooking until the liquid has completely evaporated.

3. In a blender, add in the egg whites, tofu, eggs, turmeric, black pepper, and salt. Process the ingredients until it forms a smooth mixture. When the liquid has completely evaporated from the pan, pour in the egg mixture to the spinach.

4. Remove the pan from the heat and transfer it into the oven. Bake for 25 minutes or until the eggs are set in the middle. Remove the pan from the oven and invert it on a serving plate to transfer the frittata and let stand for 10 minutes. Slice into wedges then serve.

Gluten-Free Strawberry Crepes

Ingredients:

- ✓ 6 cups of sliced strawberries
- ✓ 4 large eggs
- ✓ 2 tbsp of sugar OR honey
- ✓ 1 cup of unsweetened almond milk
- ✓ 1 tsp of vanilla extract
- ✓ 2 tbsp of light olive oil
- ✓ 1 tbsp of light brown sugar
- ✓ ¾ cup of gluten-free flour baking mix
- ✓ 1/8 tsp of salt

Procedure:

1. In a mixing bowl, combine the strawberries and sugar or honey. Let stand for 30 minutes at room temperature.

2. In a medium-sized bowl, add in the eggs, unsweetened almond milk, light olive oil, vanilla extract, light brown sugar, and salt. Whisk the ingredients together until well-incorporated. Then, add in the gluten-free flour baking mix. Continue whisking until the ingredients are properly combined.

3. Prepare an 8" nonstick skillet or crepe pan and set it over medium heat. Take ¼ cup of batter and add it into the pan. Swirl to coat the pan. Cook for 45 seconds or until the crepe is just beginning to brown. Flip and cook the other side for 10 seconds then transfer in onto a serving plate.

4. Place ½ cup of the strawberry mixture on half of the crepe then fold the crepe in half to form a semicircle. Drizzle syrup from the strawberry mixture over the crepe then serve.

Chapter 3: Lunch Recipes

Quick and Easy Pumpkin Soup

Ingredients:

- ✓ 1 cup of chopped onion

- ✓ 1 clove of garlic, minced

- ✓ 1 1" piece of gingerroot, peeled and minced

- ✓ 6 cups of vegetable stock, divided

- ✓ 1 tsp of salt

- ✓ 4 cups of pumpkin puree

- ✓ ½ tsp of fresh thyme, chopped

- ✓ 1 tsp of fresh parsley, chopped

- ✓ ½ cup of half-and-half

Procedure:

1. Prepare a large soup pot and set it over medium-high heat. Add in the onion, gingerroot, garlic, and ½ cup of vegetable stock into the pot and stir. Cook the vegetables for 5 minutes or until the vegetables are tender.

2. Add in the pumpkin puree, salt, thyme, and the remaining 5 ½ cups of vegetable stock. Stir the ingredients together and cook for 30 minutes.

3. Pour the soup in a food processor or use a handheld blender to puree the mixture until it becomes smooth.

4. Add in half-and-half into the soup and stir. Then, transfer the soup on a serving bowl and sprinkle with fresh parsley before serving.

Kippers Salad

Ingredients:

- ✓ ½ cup of reduced-fat mayonnaise
- ✓ 1 stalk of celery, finely chopped
- ✓ 1 small onion, finely chopped
- ✓ 1 tbsp of chopped fresh parsley
- ✓ 1 clove of garlic, minced
- ✓ 1 tsp of lemon juice
- ✓ 1/8 tsp of salt
- ✓ 1 (6 oz) can of kippers, drained
- ✓ 1/8 tsp of ground black pepper

Procedure:

1. In a mixing bowl, add in the mayonnaise, onion, celery, parsley, lemon juice, garlic, salt, and black pepper. Stir the ingredients together until well-incorporated. Add in the kippers and gently mix to combine. Place it inside the refrigerator until ready to use.

Roasted Chicken Wraps

Ingredients:

- ✓ ½ cup of reduced-fat mayonnaise
- ✓ 1 tsp of freshly cracked black pepper
- ✓ 2 tbsp of pickle juice
- ✓ 1 ½ cups of shredded red cabbage
- ✓ ¼ tsp of kosher salt
- ✓ 1 tbsp of apple cider vinegar
- ✓ ¼ tsp of cayenne pepper
- ✓ 6 whole wheat OR mixed grain flatbreads
- ✓ 1 deli-roasted chicken, cooled

Procedure:

1. In a large bowl, add in the mayonnaise, black pepper, and pickle juice. Stir the ingredients together until well-combined then place the bowl in the refrigerator. In another bowl, add in the red cabbage, salt, apple cider vinegar, and cayenne pepper. Toss the ingredients to combine.

2. Remove and throw away the bones and skin from the chicken then shred the meat to make bite-sized pieces. Add

the chicken pieces into the mayonnaise mixture and mix thoroughly.

3. Divide the chicken mixture and the cabbage mixture evenly among the slices of flatbreads. Roll to secure the filling and enjoy.

Persimmon and Pear Salad

Ingredients:

- ✓ 1 tsp of whole grain mustard
- ✓ 3 tbsp of extra virgin olive oil
- ✓ 2 tbsp of fresh lemon juice
- ✓ 1 shallot, minced
- ✓ 1 ripe persimmon, sliced
- ✓ 1 tsp of minced garlic
- ✓ 1 ripe red pear, sliced
- ✓ 6 cups of baby spinach
- ✓ ½ cup of chopped pecans, toasted

Procedure:

1. In a salad bowl, add in the whole grain mustard, lemon juice, olive oil, shallot, and garlic. Whisk the ingredients together until well-incorporated. Add in the persimmon, red pear, pecans, and baby spinach then toss to coat. Serve immediately.

Roasted Sweet Potato Soup

Ingredients:

- ✓ 2 ½ lbs of sweet potatoes

- ✓ ¼ tsp of kosher salt

- ✓ 1 tbsp of extra virgin olive oil

- ✓ ½ tsp of freshly cracked pepper

- ✓ 1 1" piece of ginger, peeled and minced

- ✓ 1 ½ cups of thinly sliced leeks OR onions

- ✓ 1 tsp of minced garlic

- ✓ 1 tsp of chopped fresh thyme leaves

- ✓ ½ cup of dry white wine

- ✓ 5 cups of vegetable broth

- ✓ 2 cups of orange juice

Procedure:

1. Turn on the oven and set it to 400F.

2. Remove the skins from the sweet potatoes and cut it into 1" pieces. Prepare a baking sheet and place the potatoes on it. Drizzle with olive oil and season using salt and pepper. Place the baking sheet in the oven and bake for 45 minutes

or until the sweet potatoes are well-browned and tender. Toss occasionally.

3. Prepare a large soup pot or Dutch oven and spray it with cooking spray. Set it over medium-high heat. Add in the leeks and cook for 8 minutes or until the leaves are tender and wilted. Add in the garlic and ginger and cook for 1 minute. Add in the dry white wine. Stir then bring the mixture to a boil. Continue cooking until the white wine has completely evaporated then add in the vegetable broth. Add in the thyme and sweet potatoes. Stir and bring the soup to a boil. Turn down the heat and simmer for 20 minutes or until all the vegetables are tender.

4. Pour the soup in an immersion blender and puree until it becomes smooth. Heat the soup again before serving.

Smoked Trout Tartine

Ingredients:

- ✓ 2 tbsp of freshly squeezed lemon juice
- ✓ 1 tsp of Dijon mustard
- ✓ 1 tbsp of extra virgin olive oil
- ✓ A pinch of sugar
- ✓ 2 tbsp of capers, rinsed and drained
- ✓ ¾ lb of smoked trout, flaked into bite-size pieces
- ✓ ½ cup of roasted red peppers, diced
- ✓ 1 stalk of celery, finely chopped
- ✓ ½ (15 oz) can of cannellini beans, drained and rinsed
- ✓ 2 tbsp of minced onion
- ✓ 4 large ½" thick slices of crusty whole grain bread, toasted
- ✓ 1 tsp of chopped fresh dill
- ✓ Dill sprigs

Procedure:

1. In a large bowl, add in the lemon juice, olive oil, Dijon mustard, and sugar. Whisk the ingredients together. Add in

the trout, capers, red peppers, cannellini beans, celery, onion, and dill. Toss the ingredients to combine.

2. Arrange the bread slices on a serving plate. Divide the trout mixture equally among the bread slices then place the mixture on top of the bread. Use the dill sprigs for garnish then   serve.

Lentil and Garbanzo Soup

Ingredients:

- ✓ 2 onions, chopped
- ✓ 1 cup of diced carrots
- ✓ 1 cup of chopped celery
- ✓ 2 tsp of grated fresh ginger
- ✓ 1 tsp of garam masala
- ✓ 1 tsp of minced garlic
- ✓ 1 tsp of turmeric
- ✓ ¼ tsp of ground cayenne pepper
- ✓ ½ tsp of ground cumin
- ✓ 6 cups of vegetable broth OR stock
- ✓ 2 (15 oz) cans of garbanzo beans, rinsed and drained
- ✓ 1 cup of lentils
- ✓ 1 (14.5 oz) can of petit diced tomatoes, undrained

Procedure:

1. Prepare a large soup pot and spray it with cooking spray. Set it over medium-high heat. Add in the onions and sauté for 3 minutes or until the onions are tender.

27

2. Add in the celery and carrots then cook for another 5 minutes.

3. Add in the garlic, garam masala, turmeric, cumin, and cayenne pepper. Stir and cook for 30 seconds.

4. Pour in the vegetable broth or stock and add in the lentils, garbanzo beans, and tomatoes. Stir and cook for 90 minutes or until the lentils become tender.

5. To make the soup a bit creamier and thicker, you can puree half of it and stir it back into the pot.

Chapter 4: Dinner Recipes

Poached Eggs with Curried Vegetables

Ingredients:

- ✓ 2 tsp of extra virgin olive oil
- ✓ 2 cloves of garlic, minced
- ✓ 1 large onion, chopped
- ✓ 1 tbsp of yellow curry powder
- ✓ 2 medium zucchinis, diced
- ✓ ½ lb of sliced button mushrooms
- ✓ 1 (14 oz) can of chickpeas, drained
- ✓ 1/8 tsp of crushed red pepper
- ✓ 1 cup of water
- ✓ ½ tsp of white vinegar
- ✓ 4 large eggs

Procedure:

1. Prepare a large nonstick skillet and set it over medium-high heat. Add in the onion and sauté for 4 minutes or until the onion is tender. Add in the garlic and cook for 30 seconds. Add in the curry powder and stir the ingredients together. Cook for 1 minute or until the mixture is very fragrant.

2. Add in the mushrooms and cook for 5 minutes or until the mushrooms are tender and have released all of its liquid. Add in the chickpeas, zucchini, red pepper, and water. Stir then bring the liquid to a boil. Turn down the heat and place a lid over the pan. Let it simmer for 15 minutes or until the zucchini becomes tender.

3. Prepare a large saucepan and fill it with water about 3" deep. Let it boil then turn the heat down. Add in the white vinegar and let it simmer.

4. Crack the eggs then gently slip it into the simmering liquid one at a time. Then, cook for 3 minutes or until the eggs are cooked according to your desired doneness. Remove the eggs from the hot water using a slotted spoon.

Weeknight Turkey Chili

Ingredients:

- ✓ Vegetable cooking spray
- ✓ 1 tbsp of garlic, minced
- ✓ 1 large onion, chopped
- ✓ 1 ½ lbs of ground turkey
- ✓ 1 (28 oz) can of crushed tomatoes
- ✓ 2 cups of water
- ✓ 1 (16 oz) can of kidney beans, drain then rinse
- ✓ 2 tsp of turmeric
- ✓ 2 tbsp of chili powder
- ✓ 1 tsp of smoked paprika
- ✓ 1 tsp of ground cumin
- ✓ 1 tsp of dried oregano
- ✓ 1 tsp of hot sauce

Procedure:

1. Prepare a large soup pot and spray it with vegetable cooking spray. Add in the onion and cook for 5 minutes or until the onion becomes tender and starts to brown. Add in

the garlic and cook for 30 seconds. Add in the ground turkey and cook for 10 minutes. Stir the ingredients frequently. Add in the water, tomatoes, kidney beans, chili powder, turmeric, paprika, oregano, cumin, and hot sauce. Stir the ingredients together then bring the mixture to a boil.

2. Turn the heat down and let it simmer for 30 minutes

3. .

Crusted Tilapia with Kale

Ingredients:

- ✓ ¼ cup of roasted Brazil nuts
- ✓ 2 tbsp of grated parmesan cheese
- ✓ ½ cup of fresh bread crumbs
- ✓ ¼ cup of whole grain mustard
- ✓ Vegetable cooking spray
- ✓ 1 ½ lbs of tilapia fillets
- ✓ 1 tbsp of sesame oil
- ✓ 1 ½ heads of kale, chopped
- ✓ 1 clove of garlic, mashed
- ✓ ¼ tsp of kosher salt
- ✓ 2 tbsp of toasted sesame seeds

Procedure:

1. Turn on the oven and set it to 400F. Prepare a baking sheet and spray it with vegetable cooking spray.

2. In a food processor, add in the Brazil nuts and process until the nuts are ground finely. In a small bowl, add in the ground nuts, parmesan cheese, and breadcrumbs. Stir the ingredients together until properly combined.

3. Place the tilapia fillets on the prepared baking sheet. Spread the mustard evenly on top of the fish fillets. Divide the breadcrumb mixture evenly among the fillets of fish. Spray the fish fillets with vegetable cooking spray. Place the baking pan into the oven and bake for 8 minutes or until the fish is properly cooked.

4. Prepare a large stainless steel or cast-iron skillet and set it over medium-high heat. Add in the sesame oil and wait for 15 seconds before adding in the garlic. Cook for 20 seconds then add in the kale. Cook for 7 minutes or until the kale becomes tender. Stir frequently while cooking. Add in the sesame seeds and toss the ingredients to combine.

5. Serve the fish fillets with kale on the side.

Red Pepper and Turkey Pasta

Ingredients:

- ✓ 3 large red bell peppers
- ✓ 1 large onion, chopped
- ✓ 3 tbsp of extra virgin olive oil
- ✓ 2 tsp of minced garlic
- ✓ 1 tbsp of red wine vinegar
- ✓ 2 tbsp of fresh oregano, chopped
- ✓ 2 lbs of ground turkey
- ✓ 2 lbs of cooked rigatoni

Procedure:

1. Cut the bell peppers in half. Remove the membranes and seeds then chop the peppers coarsely.

2. Prepare a Dutch oven and set it over medium heat. Add in the olive oil. Wait until the oil is hot before adding in the red bell peppers and onion. Cook for 20 minutes or until the peppers become very tender. Add in the garlic and cook for another 5 minutes.

3. Pour the mixture in a food processor or blender and process until it becomes smooth. Then, return the sauce into the pan and set it over medium-low heat. Add in the

red wine vinegar and oregano. Stir and taste. Adjust the seasonings if needed.

4. Prepare a large skillet and spray it with vegetable cooking spray. Add in the ground turkey and sauté until cooked and beginning to brown. Add in the turkey into the sauce and let it simmer for 20 minutes.

5. Place the rigatoni on a serving dish then pour the sauce over the pasta. Serve while still hot.

Steamed Salmon with Zucchini

Ingredients:

- ✓ 1 onion, thinly sliced
- ✓ 2 small zucchini, thinly sliced
- ✓ 1 lemon, thinly sliced
- ✓ 1 cup of white wine
- ✓ 4 (6 oz) fillets of salmon
- ✓ ½ cup of water
- ✓ ¼ tsp of kosher salt
- ✓ ¼ tsp of freshly ground pepper

Procedure:

1. Prepare a large Dutch oven then add in the onion, lemon, zucchini, white wine, and water.

2. Take the salmon fillets and season it using the kosher salt and freshly ground pepper. Place a steamer rack over the vegetables in the Dutch oven. Spray the rack with cooking spray. Set the Dutch oven over medium-high heat and wait for the liquid to boil.

3. Adjust the heat to medium-low and place the salmon fillets on the steamer rack. Place a lid over the Dutch oven and steam for 8 minutes or until the fillets are cooked through.

4. Remove the fish from the steamer rack and transfer the contents of the Dutch oven on a serving platter. Place the fish fillets on top of the vegetables then serve.

Black Bean and Sweet Potato Burgers with Lime Mayonnaise

Ingredients:

- ✓ ½ cup of reduced fat mayonnaise
- ✓ ½ tsp of hot sauce
- ✓ 1 lime
- ✓ Vegetable cooking spray
- ✓ 1 jalapeno, minced
- ✓ 1 small onion, chopped
- ✓ 2 tsp of ground cumin
- ✓ 2 (14.5 oz) cans of black beans, drain then rinse and mash
- ✓ 2 tsp of minced garlic
- ✓ 2 cups of grated raw sweet potato
- ✓ 1 cup of plain breadcrumbs, divided
- ✓ 1 egg, lightly beaten
- ✓ Whole wheat hamburger buns

Procedure:

1. Turn on the broiler and set it to medium-high heat. Place an oven rack about 4" to 5" from the broiler.

2. Take the zest and juice from the lime and add it into a small bowl. Add in the hot sauce and mayonnaise. Stir the ingredients together until properly combined then place the bowl in the refrigerator until needed.

3. Prepare a large skillet and set it over medium-high heat. Spray it with cooking spray then add in the onion. Cook for 4 minutes or until the onion is tender. Add in the jalapeno, garlic, and cumin. Cook for 30 seconds while stirring.

4. Transfer the onion mixture into a large bowl. Add in the sweet potato, black beans, ½ cup of breadcrumbs, and egg. Stir the ingredients together until well-combined.

5. Form the breadcrumb mixture into 8 patties and sprinkle each with the remaining breadcrumbs. Prepare a baking sheet and spray it with cooking spray. Arrange the patties on the baking sheet and spray with cooking spray.

6. Place the baking sheet into the oven and broil each side for 8 minutes or until the patties are cooked through and golden brown in color. Serve on hamburger buns with the mayonnaise mixture.

Quinoa and Turkey Stuffed Pepper

Ingredients:

- ✓ 1 cup of uncooked quinoa
- ✓ ½ tsp of salt
- ✓ 2 cups of water
- ✓ ½ lb of fully-cooked smoked turkey sausage, already diced
- ✓ ¼ cup of extra virgin olive oil
- ✓ ½ cup of chicken stock
- ✓ 3 tbsp of chopped pecans, toasted
- ✓ 2 tsp of chopped fresh rosemary
- ✓ 2 tbsp of chopped fresh parsley
- ✓ 3 red bell peppers

Procedure:

1. In a large saucepan, add in the quinoa, water, and salt. Stir the ingredients together then set the pan over high heat. Bring the mixture to a boil then adjust the heat to low. Place a lid over the saucepan and simmer for 15 minutes or until all the liquid is absorbed.

2. Remove the lid and wait for 5 minutes before adding in the turkey sausage, chicken stock, olive oil, pecans, parsley,

and rosemary. Stir the ingredients together until well-combined.

3. Cut the red bell peppers in half then remove the membranes and seeds. Boil water and cook the peppers for 5 minutes then drain.

4. Prepare a 13" x 9" baking dish and spray it with cooking spray. Arrange the pepper halves on it. Fill each pepper half with the quinoa mixture then place the baking dish in the oven once done. Bake for 15 minutes at 350F.

Chapter 5: Dessert Recipes

Nutritious Chocolate Pudding

Ingredients:

- ✓ 2 ¼ cups of milk
- ✓ ¼ cup of maple syrup
- ✓ 3 egg yolks
- ✓ ¼ cup of sucanat
- ✓ 3 tbsp of cocoa powder
- ✓ 4 tbsp of arrowroot powder
- ✓ ¼ tsp of salt
- ✓ 2 tsp of vanilla
- ✓ 3 tbsp of butter

Procedure:

1. Prepare a large saucepan and set it over medium heat. Add in the milk, maple syrup, egg yolks, sucanat, cocoa powder, arrowroot powder, and salt. Whisk the ingredients together until properly incorporated.

2. Continue stirring for 7 minutes or until the mixture becomes thick.

3. Take a spoon and dip it into the mixture. If it coats the spoon, remove the pan from the heat immediately.

4. Add in the vanilla and butter then stir to combine.

5. Pour the pudding into ramekins and serve immediately. You can also place it in the refrigerator if you prefer cold chocolate pudding.

No Bake Cookie Bars

Ingredients:

- ✓ 1 cup of natural peanut butter

- ✓ ½ cup of organic coconut oil

- ✓ ½ cup of honey

- ✓ 2 cups of organic dry oats

- ✓ 1 cup of chopped pecans

- ✓ 1 cup of unsweetened coconut flakes, already shredded

- ✓ 1 ¼ cups of dark chocolate chips

Procedure:

1. Prepare a 9" x 13" baking pan and lightly grease it with coconut oil.

2. In a large bowl, add in the dry oats, pecans, coconut flakes, and chocolate chips. Stir the ingredients together until properly combined.

3. Prepare a small saucepan and add in the coconut oil, peanut butter, and honey. Place the pan over low heat and stir the ingredients together. Wait until the coconut oil has mostly melted before removing the pan from the heat.

4. Pour the honey mixture into the bowl with the oats mixture and stir until the ingredients are well-incorporated and the chocolate chips have melted completely.

5. Place the mixture onto the baking pan and spread it evenly.

6. Cover the baking pan with cling wrap and place it inside the refrigerator until the mixture has set.

7. Cut it into bars and serve.

Rustic Bread Pudding

Ingredients:

For the Pudding

- ✓ 2 cups of raw whole milk
- ✓ 2/3 cup of sucanat
- ✓ ¼ cup of pastured butter
- ✓ 3 pastured eggs
- ✓ ¼ tsp of ground nutmeg
- ✓ 2 tsp of cinnamon
- ✓ 1 tsp of vanilla extract
- ✓ ½ cup of raisins
- ✓ 3 cups of sourdough bread, torn into bite-size pieces

For the Sauce

- ✓ 1 cup of half-and-half
- ✓ 1 tsp of vanilla
- ✓ 1/8 cup of sucanat
- ✓ A dash of salt

Procedure:

1. For the sauce: Prepare a saucepan then add in the half-and-half, sucanat, vanilla, and salt. Set the pan over medium heat. Stir for 5 minutes then set it aside until needed.

2. For the pudding: Prepare a saucepan then add in the butter. Wait for the butter to melt completely before adding in the milk. Stir to combine.

3. In a mixing bowl, combine the eggs, sucanat, nutmeg, cinnamon, and vanilla. Whisk the ingredients together until well-combined then gradually add in the milk mixture. Stir the ingredients to combine.

4. Prepare a 1 ½-quart casserole dish and spray it with cooking spray. Place the bread into the dish.

5. Sprinkle the raisins over the bread then pour the mixture on top.

6. Place the casserole dish in the oven and bake for 45 minutes at 350F. Pour the sauce over the pudding once done baking then serve.

Pumpkin Coconut Fudge Squares

Ingredients:

- ✓ 1 can of pumpkin puree
- ✓ 16 dates
- ✓ 2 (200g) packs of coconut butter
- ✓ 1 tsp of cinnamon
- ✓ 1 tsp of vanilla
- ✓ 1 tsp of mixed spice
- ✓ A pinch of sea salt

Procedure:

1. Prepare a bowl of water then add in the dates. Place the bowl in the microwave oven and heat the dates for a couple of minutes until it becomes soft.

2. Place the dates in a food processor and process until it forms a goopy paste.

3. Prepare bowl of hot water and place the coconut butter packs in it. Wait until the coconut butter completely melts before removing the packs from the bowl.

4. In a mixing bowl, add in the pumpkin puree, coconut butter, date paste, cinnamon, mixed spice, vanilla, and sea salt. Stir the ingredients together until it forms a soft ball.

5. Prepare a baking tray and line it with wax paper. Spread the mixture evenly on top of the tray to make ½" thick fudge cake. Sprinkle with extra cinnamon on top then place the tray in the refrigerator until the cake hardens.

6. Cut the fudge cake into squares once set then serve.

Strawberry Gelato

Ingredients:

- ✓ 2 cups of milk

- ✓ 4 egg yolks

- ✓ 1 cup of heavy cream

- ✓ ½ cup of raw honey OR maple syrup

- ✓ ¼ tsp of sea salt

- ✓ 2 cups of fresh strawberries, remove the top part and stems then puree

- ✓ ½ tsp of lemon zest

Procedure:

1. Add in the cream and milk into a saucepan. Stir then bring the mixture to boil. Turn down the heat and simmer for 4 minutes while stirring constantly.

2. In a blender, add in the honey, salt, and egg yolks. Blend until the mixture becomes creamy and smooth.

3. Set the blender on low speed then gradually add in the warm milk into the blender. Perform this step very slowly to prevent the hot milk from cooking the eggs.

4. Return the mixture into the saucepan and adjust the heat to medium-low. Cook for 10 minutes while stirring constantly or until the mixture begins to thicken.

5. Add in the lemon zest and strawberry puree into the pan. Stir the ingredients to combine.

6. Place the mixture in the refrigerator for 4 hours or until the mixture has cooled completely. Once cool, freeze the mixture for 2 hours then add it into the blender to process until it becomes smooth. Replace the mixture into the freezer and wait for another 3 hours or until the mixture hardens. Serve and enjoy.

Conclusion

Thank you again for purchasing this book!

I hope this book was able to help you to start a healthier lifestyle beginning with your diet.

The next step is to apply and incorporate these recipes into your diet plan so you can gradually adjust your appetite to this diet.

Finally, please remember to check out our Facebook page in order to find other resources and upcoming promotions:

https://www.facebook.com/joypublishing

With sincere thanks,

Emma Rose

Emma Rose

Preview Of "Paleo Free Diet Guide for Beginners: Over 50 Paleo Diet Recipes for Fast Weight Loss and Optimal Health"

Introduction

I want to thank you and congratulate you for purchasing the book, *"Paleo Free Diet Guide for Beginners: Over 50 Paleo Diet Recipes for Optimal Health and Fast Weight Loss"*.

This book contains everything you might need to know when it comes to getting started with the Paleo diet. It is provided in an easily digestible format that allows you to better absorb the information. There are no complicated explanations about how it works! You'll be given what you need straight up so you won't have to waste time trying to understand exactly what the diet is. Whether it's for your overall good health or to lose a few pounds, Paleo can certainly help you with it. To help you get started, we'll do the same and start you off with 50 of the best Paleo recipes that you can slowly but surely shift your everyday menu to.

It's never easy changing a diet. I often fall into self pity when I can no longer have the foods I enjoy. Either I feel sorry for myself or I get rebellious and binge and anything and everything. I always knew the value of eating healthy. I could just never bring myself to do it. It wasn't until I had a miscarriage that I got serious about my health. I have made drastic changes that others just don't understand. But the pay off is the weight I've lost and the better health I'm experiencing.

My hope for you is not to be on another "diet." This isn't a restriction diet like Atkins. The goal is to have a lifestyle change. Lifestyle changes are more sustainable and maintain weight loss long term compared to restriction diets. The change is hard to start but worth it when you commit. The trick is to get the momentum to start.

Thanks again for purchasing this book. I hope you enjoy reading it and eating the recipes from it!

With gratitude,

Emma   Rose

Chapter 1 – What Is the Paleo Diet?

The Paleo Diet is known by many names such as the cavemen diet, stone age diet and hunter-gatherer diet, to name a few. The concept behind this diet follows that of the Paleolithic era before the development of agriculture. Essentially, you consume the same foods that the cavemen used to eat. The focus is on eating food closest to its natural, unprocessed state. The cavemen would gather their food from any source available whether it was wild animals, berries, vegetables, or fruits. As a result, they were strong, fit, and healthy for thousand of years.

This type of diet is still very young, less than fifty years only, but more in depth researches and studies are being conducted to increase the information and knowledge on this diet. The results of previous studies conducted on the Paleo diet reveal the improvement of health to the people involved. This is attributed to the fact that no processed foods and additives are included. The Paleo Diet is a diet that works with our genetics – before machinery and processing got involved. Foods that were not available during the Paleolithic time such as dairy products, salt, sugar and grains are not included in the preparation of the Paleo diet.

The modern diet predominately consumed in the Western world is full of refined foods, trans fats, salt and sugar. These ingredients are known to indirectly cause diseases such as hypertension, diabetes, strokes, obesity and other heart problems. The list goes on even further with the increase diagnosis of cancer, Parkinson's, Alzheimer's, depression and infertility. "What an extraordinary achievement for a civilization: to have developed the one diet that reliably makes its people sick!" (Michael Pollen, Food Rules: An Eater's Manual, Penguin Books 2009).

Foods included in the Paleo Diet

- Fruit

- Vegetables

- Lean Meat

- Seafood

- Nuts/Seeds

- Healthy Fats (eg. coconut, avocado, nuts and seeds, olive oil, grass fed butter)

Foods NOT included in the Paleo Diet

- Dairy

- Grain

- Processed Food

Why not grain?

You may be surprised to see that grains are not included in the Paleo Diet. We are accustomed to grains being a part of a balanced diet. However, our bodies are not designed to deal with the nutritional components of grains such as gluten, lectin, and phytates.

Gluten is a protein substance found in wheat, barley and rye. Many people are discovering that their bodies are gluten sensitive and are eliminating gluten from their diet. The most extreme case of gluten sensitivity is Celiac Disease. Individuals with this disease can pick up the minutest trace of gluten and react immediately.

Lectin binds to insulin receptors and can also cause leptin resistance.

Phytates cause minerals to become unavailable during digestion.

Why is dairy a problem?

When purchasing milk, you need to be mindful of the source.

Check out the rest of "Paleo Free Diet Guide for Beginners: Over 50 Paleo Diet Recipes for Fast Weight Loss and Optimal Health" on Amazon

Or go to: http://amzn.to/1jIJUFX

Check Out My Other Books

Below you'll find some of my other books also available on Amazon and Kindle. Search for these titles on the Amazon website to find them.

Paleo Free Diet Guide for Beginners: Over 50 Paleo Free Recipes for Optimal Health & Fast Weight Loss

Paleo Desserts: Satisfy Your Sweet Tooth With Over 100 Quick & Easy Paleo Dessert Recipes & Paleo Baking Recipes

Raw Food Diet Guide: Lose Weight Quickly, Achieve Optimal Health & Feel Energized with the Raw Food Diet & Raw Food Recipes

Clean Eating Guide: Lose Weight Quickly, Achieve Optimal Health & Feel Energized with Clean Eating For Busy Families & Clean Eating Recipes

Alkaline Diet Guide: Lose Weight Quickly, Achieve Optimal Health & Feel Energized with the Alkaline Diet & Alkaline Recipes

Coconut Flour Recipes for Optimal Health & Quick Weight Loss: Gluten Free Recipes for Celiac Disease, Gluten Sensitivities & Paleo Free Diets

Almond Flour Recipes for Optimal Health & Quick Weight Loss: Gluten Free Recipes for Celiac Disease, Gluten Sensitivities & Paleo Free Diets

Wheat Free Diet for Beginners: Lose Weight Quickly, Achieve Optimal Health & Feel Energized with Gluten Free Recipes for Celiac Disease, Gluten Sensitivities & Paleo Free Diets

Detox Diet Guide: Lose Weight Quickly, Achieve Optimal Health & Feel Energized Through the 10 Day Detox

Sugar Detox Guide for Beginners: Lose Weight Quickly, Achieve Optimal Health, Feel Energized & Eliminate Sugar Cravings Naturally

Ketogenic Diet Guide for Beginners: How to Achieve Rapid Weight Loss, Optimal Health & Unstoppable Energy with Ketogenic Diet Recipes

Anti Inflammatory Diet for Beginners: Lose Weight Fast, Optimize Health, Slow Aging, Fight Inflammation, Conquer Pain & Increase Energy with the Anti Inflammation Diet Recipes

One Last Thing...

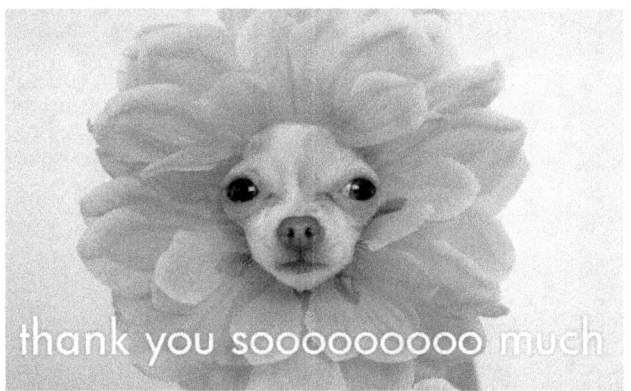

thank you soooooooooo much

If you believe that this book is worth sharing, would you please take the time to let others know how it affected your life? If it turns out to make a difference in the lives of others, they will be forever grateful to you, as will I.